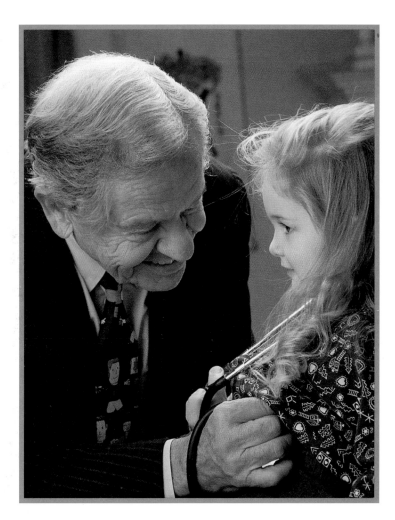

Going to the Doctor

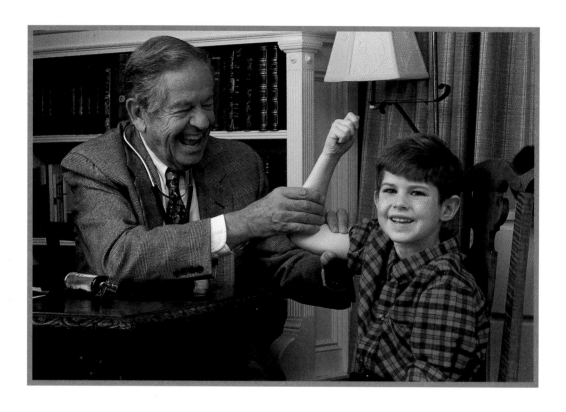

A Merloyd Lawrence Book

✦Addison-Wesley Publishing Company, Inc.

Reading, Massachusetts • Menlo Park, California
New York • Don Mills, Ontario • Harlow, England
Amsterdam • Bonn • Sydney • Singapore
Tokyo • Madrid • San Juan • Paris • Seoul
Milan • Mexico City • Taipei

Going to the Doctor

T. Berry Brazelton, M.D.

Drawings by Alfred Womack
Photographs by Sam Ogden

Library of Congress Cataloging-in-Publication Data

Brazelton, T. Berry, 1918–
    Going to the Doctor / T. Berry Brazelton ; drawings by Alfred Womack ; photographs by Sam Ogden.
      p.   cm.
    "A Merloyd Lawrence Book."
    Summary: A pediatrician tells what happens when a child goes to the doctor for a checkup, with explanations of the instruments and procedures that will be encountered.
    ISBN 0-201-40694-2
    1. Children--medical examinations--Juvenile literature.
2. Children--preparation for medical care--Juvenile literature.
[1. Medical care. 2. Children's art.] I. Womack, Alfred, ill.
II. Ogden, Sam, ill. III. Title.
RJ50.5.B73   1996
618.92'0075--dc20   96-9000
                                      CIP
                                      AC

Jacket design by Suzanne Heiser
Text design and composition by Amy R. Bernstein
Border design by Pamela Levy
Set in 16/22-point Simoncini Garamond

1 2 3 4 5 6 7 8 9-RNV-0099989796
First printing, August 1996

For Max

Acknowledgements

As I explain in the afterword, this book is the idea of six-year-old Max Dower of Los Angeles. He challenged me to try writing for children for the first time. I am indebted to him and to his perceptive mother, Kim Dower, who saw the need for a book on going to the doctor that empathizes with the child's feelings and made sure that neither I nor my friend and editor, Merloyd Lawrence, nor my publisher, Addison-Wesley, forgot this challenge! I hope that Max and all inquiring children like him will find that the text and my grandson Alfred's pictures understand their concerns and explain the reasons for each part of a visit to the doctor or nurse practitioner. We want to make the visit the rewarding event it can be.

The sensitive and lovely photographs by Sam Ogden make vividly clear what we try to accomplish in a checkup. Sam's son, Evan, is one of our delightful "models" and lured me into a strenuous game of peekaboo.

My colleague Casey Schwartz has been her usual invaluable self, as she contacted the brave and wonderful children in the photographs. Constance Keefer, M.D., one of my cherished pediatric colleagues, kindly checked the text for accuracy.

I am indebted to them all.

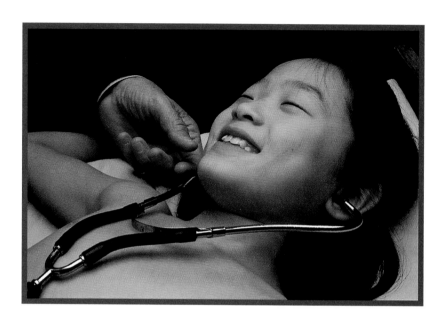

Contents

Introduction 9

Your Own Doctor 10

Talking to Your Doctor 12

Getting Undressed 14

Your Heart and Lungs 16

Your Throat 18

Your Ears 20

Your Belly 22

Your Private Parts 24

Your Nerves and Muscles 26

Your Weight and Height 28

Your Blood Pressure 30

Your Eyes 32

Shots 34

Medicines 36

All Done! 38

Afterword for Parents 40

Sample Questions for Parents to Ask 47

About the Author, Illustrator, and Photographer 48

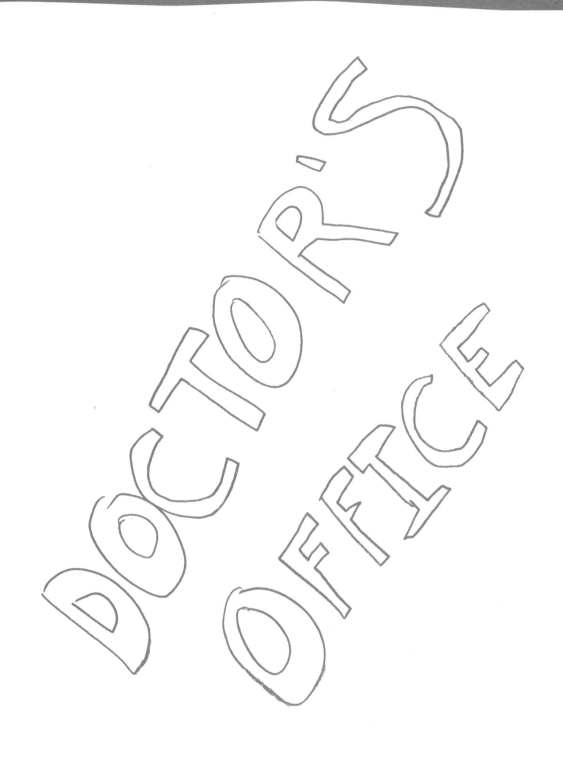

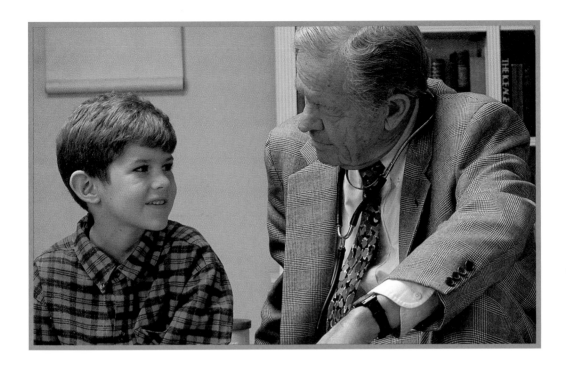

Introduction

Have you ever wondered why your parents bring you to the doctor for a "checkup" even when you're not sick? Will you get shots? Or is the visit just to be sure you're okay? Will you have to go again next year?

Since I'm a doctor who takes care of children, I've written this book to answer your questions and let you know what the doctor is looking for.

The drawings are by my nine-year-old grandson. He wanted to let me know how each part of the visit to his doctor felt to him. Maybe you'll agree.

Your Own Doctor

A doctor who takes care of kids is called a pediatrician. Let's pretend I'm yours. When you come to see me, I want to make sure you are healthy. I also want to help you learn how to take care of yourself, so that when you grow up you can get away from all of us nosy adults. I weigh and measure you, listen to you, and poke you to see whether everything's where it ought to be. I want to know how you're doing at school, with your family, and with your friends. I enjoy getting to know you better each visit. Your parents will have questions about you. Embarrassing, aren't they?

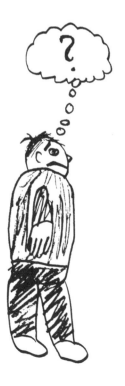 I also like to talk to you by yourself. It may make you feel weird to be with me all alone, but it helps me get to know *you* as a person. As you get older, if you have worries, I can be one you talk to.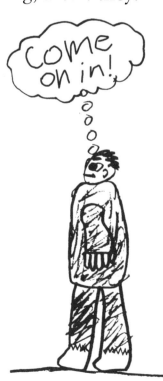

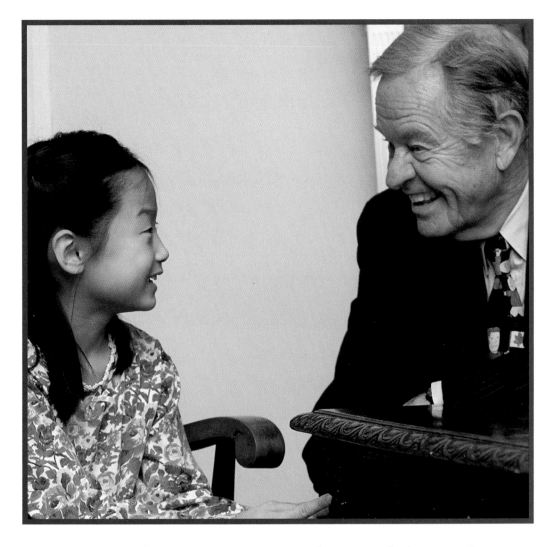

For I'm *your* doctor, not your mother's or father's. They have their own.

Some children see a special kind of nurse called a "pediatric nurse practitioner" when they go for their checkups. The nurse will examine you in much the same way that I describe in this book.

Talking to Your Doctor

After I've sat and talked to your parents, it's time for me to talk to you. I've watched your face for signals, since I know some children are worried about coming to me and it's hard to speak up. Do you know how I can tell? When you like what we're saying, your whole face brightens, your eyebrows go up, and you almost smile. When we're talking

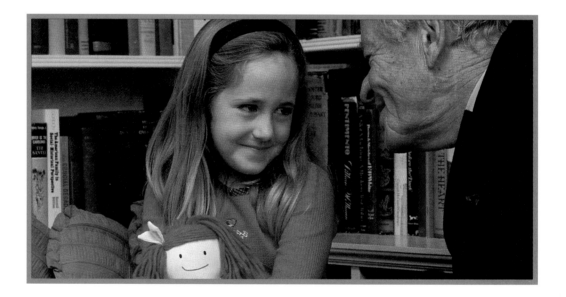

about you and you disagree or are embarrassed, your face gets dark. Your eyes get cloudy or glum, and your body gets tense. I wish I could hear what you're thinking. Not that either of us would disagree with your parents, because we know they care so much about you. But you might have

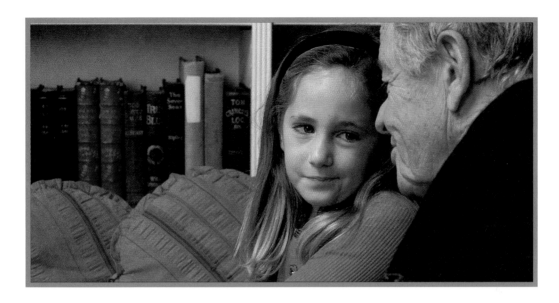

other ideas, and I'd like to know about them.

When it's time for me to examine you, I'll ask how you want to do it. Should I ask your parents to leave the room so you can have privacy? Or would you rather keep them there for protection? When you were a baby, I used to examine you in your mother's lap, because I knew how scary it was to come to the doctor, to have to undress, and to have me use all my strange instruments. Your mother or father might want to stay in the room. They probably don't want to miss any comments you or I might have.

13

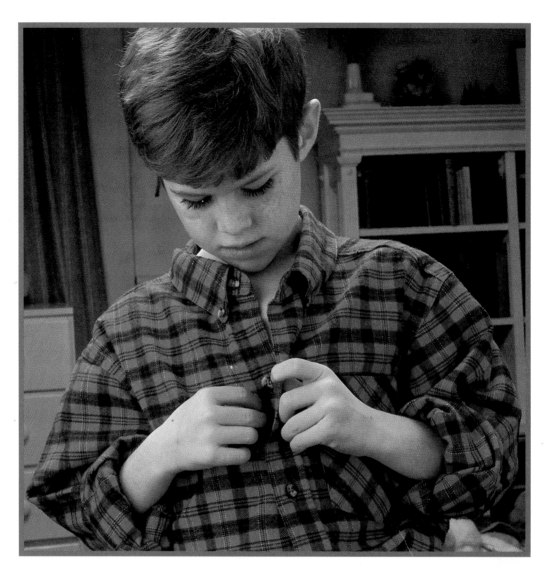

Getting Undressed

I know that getting undressed in a strange place is one of the most embarrassing things I can ask of you. So, take your time. And keep your underpants on. If I need to check underneath them, I can do it without your taking them off. I'm sure that will feel better.

First, I watch how you stand. Is your back straight? Are your legs and feet straight? Are they the same length? A few kids have one leg shorter than the other when they are beginning to grow fast. As I look you over quickly, I'm checking on a few things like that, but I don't want to make you stay bare for too long.

As you climb on the examining table, I'm watching how your muscles work. You are beginning to get some muscles, and they are going to be powerful. I also check your skin all over for any rashes.

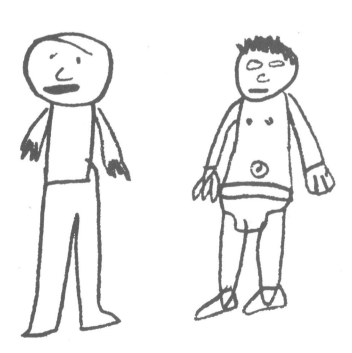

Your Heart and Lungs

Have you ever listened through a stethoscope? It makes the sounds from your body louder. The first touch on your chest might feel cold, but after that it warms up on your skin. Let me know if you'd like to listen, too, or try it on your daddy or mommy.

Your heart makes two sounds close together (boom-blub, boom-blub). One sound, "boom," is the heart pumping blood into your lungs through a special little door called a valve. The blood picks up oxygen to carry all through your

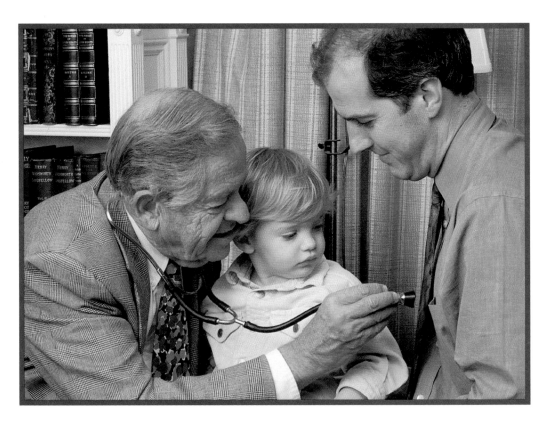

body. (If you've been running, your heart beats faster. I can hear that through my stethoscope.)

The heart opens up to let the blood back in through another little valve. When that valve closes, it makes the second sound, "blub." The heart is filled up and ready to pump again, boom-blub, boom-blub. If I heard anything different, I'd explain what I heard.

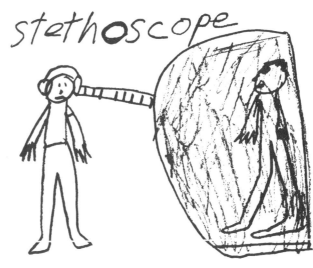

stethoscope

After I listen to your heart, I listen to your lungs. Have you heard wind sighing in and out of a door that was opening and closing slightly? That's what your breath sounds like—breathing in and breathing out. I'm listening for wheezes when you breathe out (asthma sounds like that), or crackles (pneumonia sounds like Rice Krispies), or wheezes when your breath goes in (which could be croup or bronchitis). If you had any of these, you'd probably feel sick or feverish, and I would want to know about it. My grandson thinks the stethoscope feels like it's swallowing his whole body. How does it feel to you?

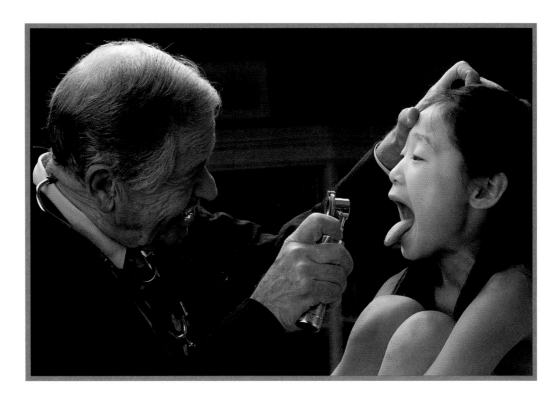

Your Throat

When I say the word "doctor" to my two-year-old grand-
daughter, Rosie, she pulls up her shirt and opens her mouth
wide. She knows just what I do.

If you can open your mouth wide and say "Ah-h,"
I won't need to use a tongue depressor—a throat stick—
to see in there. I want to see your tonsils and all of your
tongue. Tonsils are red patches on the sides of your throat,
way back. Sometimes they get very big and have white
patches on them. That's when your throat is sore. I may

look at your teeth and make sure your gums are healthy.

Next, I feel for glands in your neck. If they were swollen, they'd be the size of big marbles along your neck and under your jaw. They'd also be big if you had a bad throat infection. When there is nothing the matter, I can hardly feel them. Can you feel them?

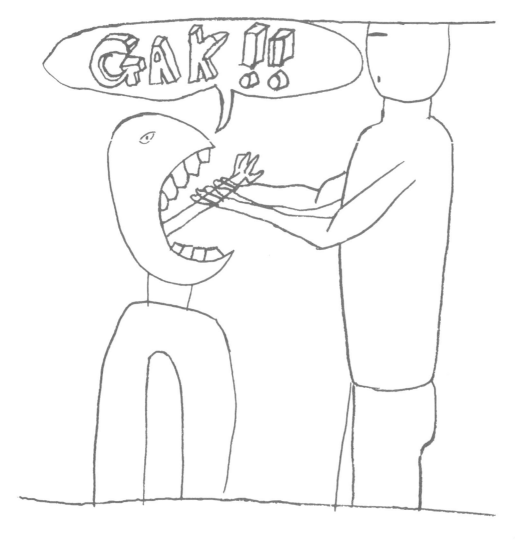

Your Ears

I always let older children look in my ear when I check theirs. One smart seven-year-old chirped up as she looked in, "Hey, I can see straight through to the other side!"

Using a metal tube with a light in it, called an otoscope, I can see into your ears. The little light makes it possible for me to see all the way to your eardrum. If you have too much wax in your ear canal, I can't see the eardrum. If that happens, I ask your mother to put some drops in before

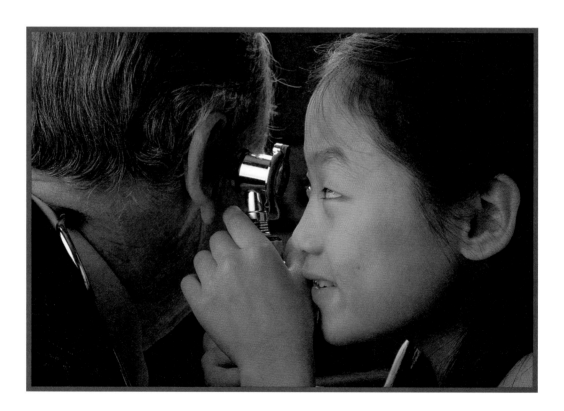

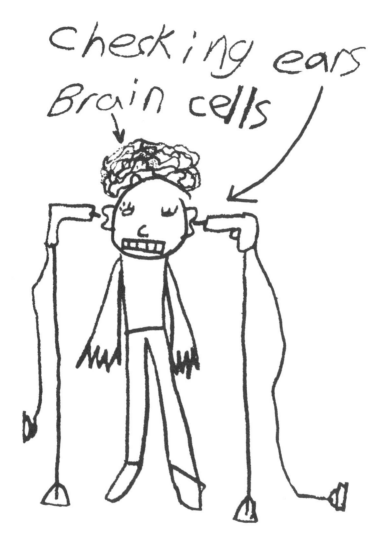

checking ears

Brain cells

you come. Then I can see the eardrum better. It is usually shiny and light pink. When you have an earache, it is swollen and red and hurts, because the infection is pressing on the eardrum from the inside. We have medicine to fix the infection and make your ear feel better.

Your Belly

If you'd rather have me check your belly when you are sitting on your parent's lap, I can. But if you climb up on the table and lie down, it's easier for me to feel everything. On the right side, I can feel your liver, underneath your ribs. Your liver helps clean your blood. On the left is your spleen, and I can't feel that at all unless it's very swollen. The spleen also helps clean your blood. Your blood needs to be pure, with new blood cells to carry oxygen and food around your body.

Some children don't like this part of the checkup at all. One little girl made her stomach all hard and turned away. When I asked why, she said she was afraid I'd feel the forbidden candy she'd eaten before she came.

Now I really get down to business, pressing hard all through your tummy to be sure everything is working right. If you had a pain or a sore spot in your belly, I'd have to figure out why. When I press, I hear a lot of gurgles. These are good. If I can't hear them, I

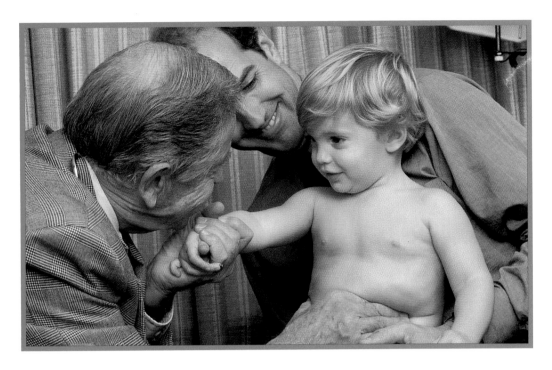

poke again and they start up, because your intestines think my pressing hand is food ready to go through them. Your intestines are like a long tube—as long as half a soccer field—all curled up! As they gurgle, they move food from where you've swallowed it, bit by bit, sopping it up to feed your body. The food that your intestines can't use becomes a BM (poop). When you are constipated (which means you haven't done a poop in a few days), I can even feel a big, hard BM in there. Little creatures called bacteria live in there and help your body use the food. Your farts are a mixture of swallowed air and the gas made by these bacteria. That's why they smell so bad.

Your Private Parts

Now comes a part of the checkup that no one likes—checking your private parts. I have to pull down your underwear for a quick look.

   If you are a boy, I need to check your penis and your testicles. If your penis had an infection, it would itch and burn when you peed. I check for redness or swelling. I check for a swelling right in the crease between your leg and body. You get a swelling here, called a hernia, if your muscles don't quite hold your intestines. It can be fixed by an awfully easy operation (but who wants an operation at all?).

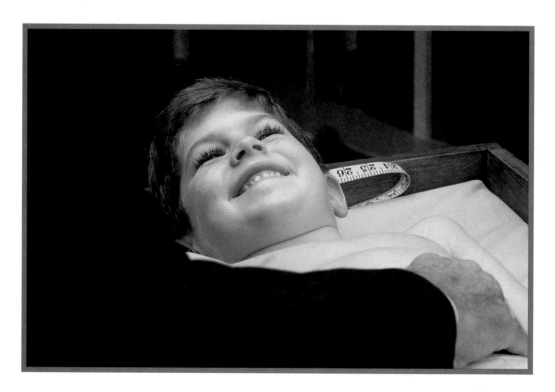

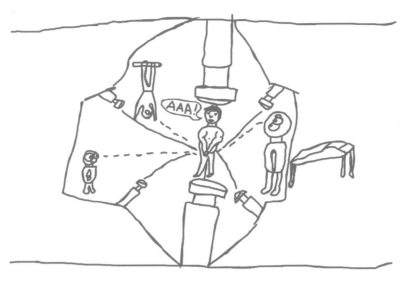

If you are a girl, I need to check your vagina and the opening where you pee to be sure they are not red and sore. If they were, it would hurt to pee and there would be a smelly spot on your underpants. We could give you medicine to clear that up.

When I get you to turn over, lying down facing the wall, I'm checking your butt (anus). If you had a swelling or sore spot around the butt, I'd hope to find it and to tell you how to fix it. Kids joke about this part of the checkup because nobody likes it.

Whether you are a boy or a girl, this exam of your private parts takes very little time at all. Unless I find a problem, it's over before you know it. Still, this part of your visit may make you shy or nervous. Don't worry. Everyone feels that way. Even grown-ups.

Your Nerves and Muscles

On some visits, I check your reflexes. I use a soft rubber hammer and hit you gently just below your knees and elbows. Your legs and arms jump when I hit a tendon that

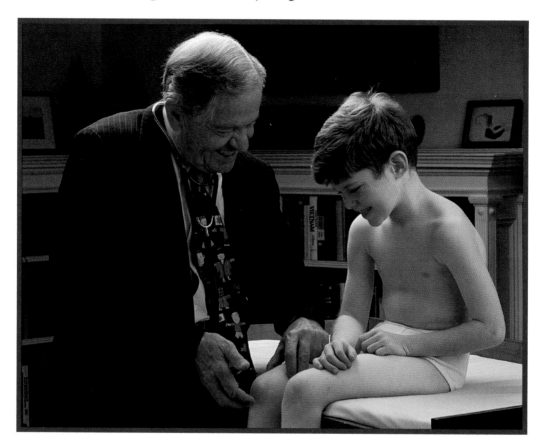

holds those joints together. When they jump, I know your nerves are okay.

Then, I do your feet. When I stroke the soles of your feet, it tickles. There is a reflex on your feet called a

Babinski reflex. It makes your toes curl up. Sometimes I do this to you to show off. It's always a funny feeling to have your body do things that you don't expect. I like to surprise you. My grandson doesn't think reflexes are funny. He says the hammer I use is as big as a rock pounder. Doesn't that show you how kids have different ideas about everything doctors do?

When you climb off the table and stand up, I watch to see how strong your muscles are. When you lean over, I can check how straight your backbone is. If you are a boy, when you are standing I have to pull your underpants down and feel for a hernia again. When you stand, your intestine pushes down into your groin (between your belly and the top of your leg), and I might see a hernia that I'd never find any other way. Sometimes I ask you to cough to put more pressure on it.

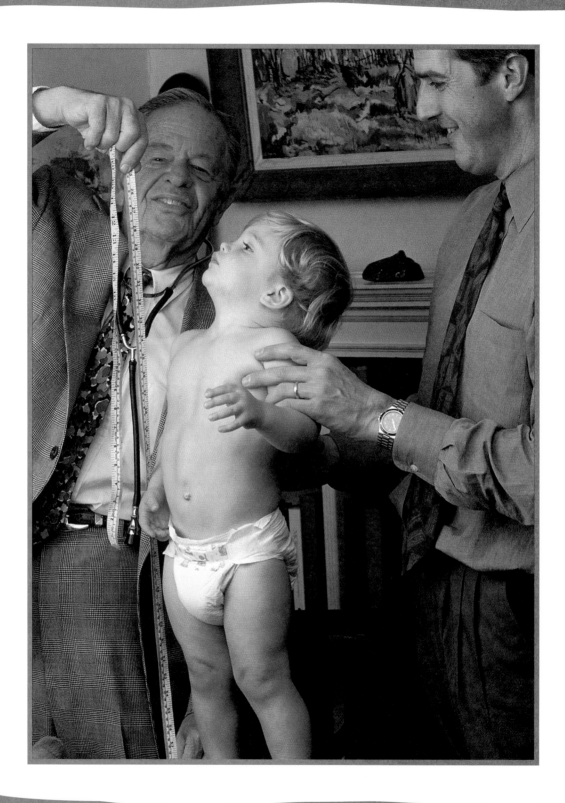

Your Weight and Height

Sometime during your visit, I weigh you and measure you. I want to see that you are growing well for your age. You'll usually grow about two inches and four or five pounds between visits until you get to be a teenager. Then you'll start stretching out and shooting up even faster. Many children worry about the shape of their bodies and whether they are too fat or too thin. I used to worry about my little brother because he was shaped like a diamond. No one always feels good about how they look. We often wish we looked like someone else. Some want more muscles. Some want to be taller, some thinner. Kids with beautiful

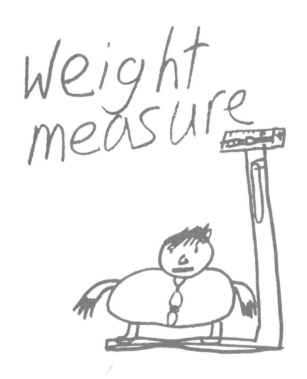

curly hair want straight hair, and so on. But usually people stop caring and really get to like the way they are.

Your Blood Pressure

Now we take your blood pressure. Do you know what blood pressure measures? The dial attached to the armband that I put on you to squeeze your upper arm is going to tell me two numbers. I listen with my stethoscope to your pulse, the heartbeat in your arm. I pump a little rubber balloon on the armband until it stops the blood flowing in your arm. Then I slowly let the air out. When I hear your blood come pounding through, I look at the needle on the

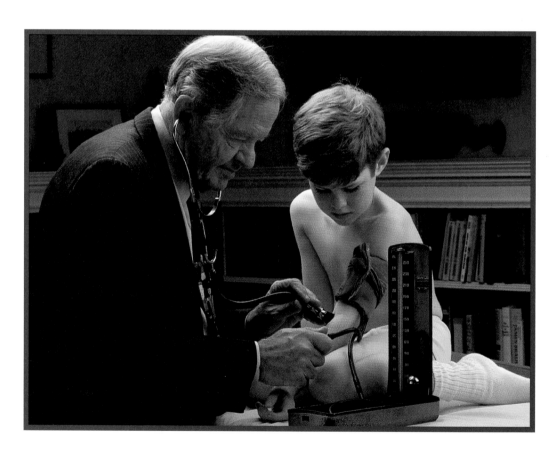

dial that tells me the first number. When you are excited or when you've been running, that number might be higher. Then I listen for another change in the sound I'm hearing. The blood sounds get very soft. I look at the dial for the second number. If that number were high, I'd be worried.

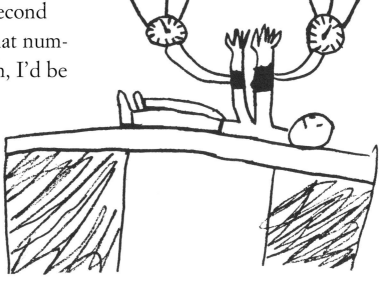

Children almost never have high blood pressure, but lots of grown-ups do. Then they need to be extra careful about what they eat (no junk food!). The reason I want to know about yours is to be able to tell if it changes later on. I'll probably remind you to eat healthy foods. My grandson says, "When you're a kid, you can eat some junk food, but not all the time." You may not listen to me, but I want you to learn how to take care of yourself as you grow and get older.

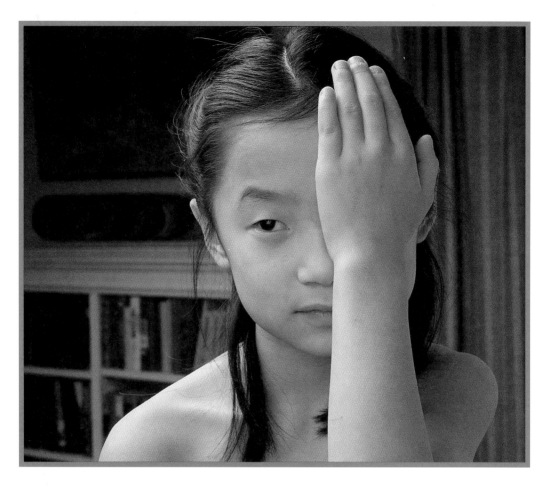

Your Eyes

Next, I check your eyes. You stand twenty feet from the eye chart and cover one eye at a time. Then you look at the pictures or letters on the chart. In some doctors' offices, children look into a machine instead. You start with big pictures or letters. Then you go down row by row. If you can read the tiny row, called row 20, with each eye, you won't need glasses. Then we say your eyesight is 20/20.

My eye chart has letters for older children and pictures for younger children who don't read yet. When I ask chil-

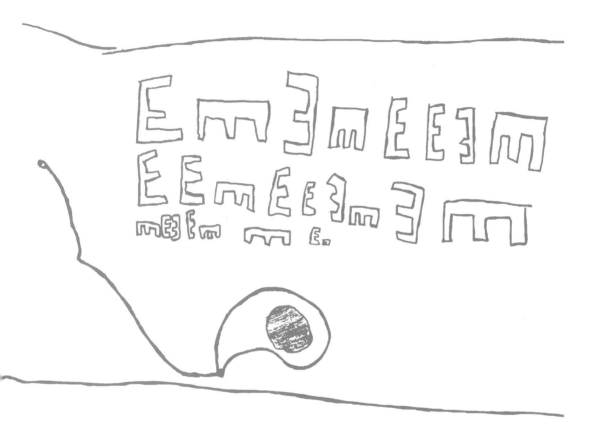

dren about the bottom rows, I get funny answers some-times. One four-year-old looked at the picture of a ship and said, "That's a lamp from my room!"

Shots

At your age, you won't need a shot at every visit. Sometimes doctors give you a test for a sickness called TB
(tuberculosis), a coughing lung disease. For that, we use an
instrument with four tiny points on it. If you get a swelling
later where we pricked your arm, it means you could have
gotten close to someone with TB. It doesn't necessarily
mean you have it, and we'll know how to cure you even if
you do. You can tell what my grandson thinks of prickly
tests by his picture of teeth about to eat him up.

Once in a while we might take a drop of blood to test.
This can be scary, but it doesn't hurt very much. Do you

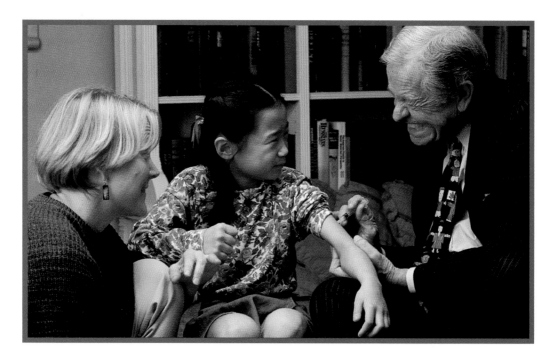

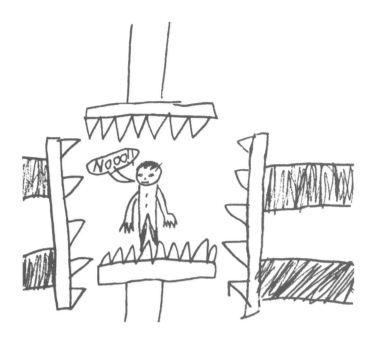

want to look? Some kids don't like to look at even a tiny drop of blood, and some yell because it might hurt. All this sounds worse than the real thing, but you probably won't believe it until afterwards. I get you to squeeze my hand or your parent's very hard to distract you while we prick your finger.

If you need any shots to keep you from getting sick, you may feel the same way. The idea of a needle stick is always worse than the moment I stick you. Hang on tight to your parents, and let out a yell if you want to. That will keep it from feeling so bad. Many kids are surprised when it is over so quickly and tell me it's no big deal.

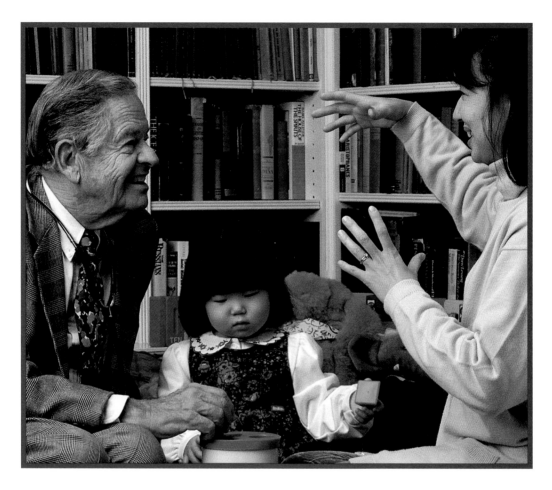

Medicines

Sometimes, if you come for a visit about a sore throat or a bad cut or an earache, I give your parent a prescription. A prescription is a note for the drugstore saying what pills or other medicine you need. You take the note to the drugstore and buy the medicine. Often children need a medicine called an antibiotic, which fights the germs that give you earaches and infections. Medicine is usually easy to take, but you and your parents have to remember! Maybe you could make a picture like this to put on the fridge.

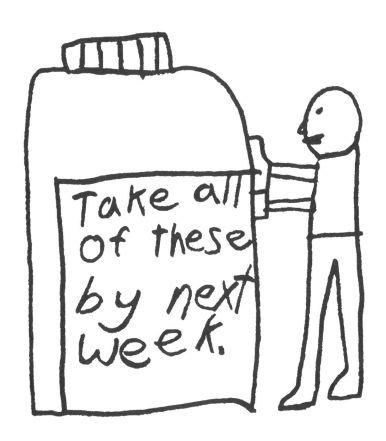

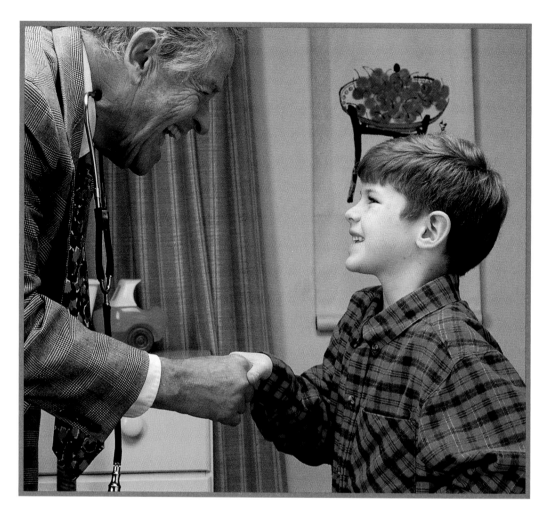

All Done!

At the end of the visit, I have a chat with you and your
parents about the ways you can stay healthy—about good
food, exercise, and plenty of sleep. When you hear this
conversation, you know the visit is almost over and that
the rest is good news!

I like to give children a reward for coming and for being so brave. It could be stickers or some other treat. I can remember all too well how worried I used to be—and still am—when I go to my doctor. It's a lot harder when you're a kid and you

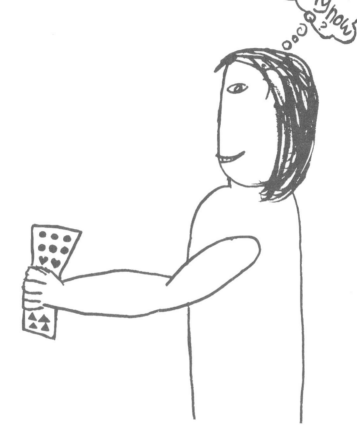

wonder why you need to go, when nothing is wrong with you. The reward is my way of telling you that your family and I are really proud of you for coming and listening and being brave. We are also very happy when you are healthy!

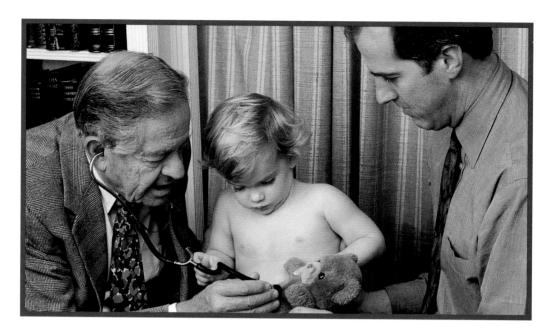

Afterword for Parents

This book owes its existence to six-year-old Max of Los Angeles. We became friends thanks to Max's mother, the publicist Kim Dower (Kim from LA), who introduced my book *Touchpoints* to a West Coast audience. One day Max joined us on a visit to the MGM studios. As we explored together, Max spotted a fascinating old monoplane. He trusted me enough to let me put him up on the wing. I climbed up beside him for a chat. "Dr B.," he said, "Why don't you write a book for kids? You always write them for grown-ups."

I was flabbergasted, and flattered. "What would I write about?" "Lots," said Max. "Write why I go to the doctor." Then he asked me a question that I will always remember. "What are you looking for when you check children? Are you looking for their badness?" This question held such insight into the reasons that children worry about a doctor's visit that I felt I must reply. This book is my explanation for Max. I hope he will approve.

I did have doubts. Writing for children daunted me. It took me years to find a voice that reaches parents. Although I talk to children all the time in my office, writing for them seemed a whole new realm. I decided to ask my nine-year-old grandson to help. "Would you write a book with me?" He looked skeptically at me. Was this homework in disguise? "I don't write," he announced. Later, when a colleague of mine, Kathryn Barnard, was visiting, she suggested that Alfred draw pictures of what it feels like to visit the doctor. Alfred started to draw, and the book began. When I read him what I wrote to go with the pictures he'd drawn, he said, "Just to be honest, Bapa, the best thing about this book will be the pictures."

Children deserve to understand why they need to be dragged into their doctor's office for checkups and immunizations. They deserve to understand the doctor's and nurse practitioner's point of view in trying to prevent future illness. Children are capable of turning this understanding into responsibility for their health. I am convinced that even small children benefit from learning how their bodies work. As one three-year-old said after she'd heard me tell her mother, who had been trying unsuccessfully to potty train her, to leave her training to her, "Dr. B. said leave it to me. I can do it!" Left alone, she did.

A sense of responsibility for one's own health begins with mutual respect between a caregiver and a child. When physicians and nurse practitioners acknowledge and work with the child's defenses against being examined, they are teaching self-respect. We are all concerned these days about molestation and about how to prepare children to avoid creepy adults. When we as physicians respect children's privacy and their bodies' intactness, as we approach them slowly and on their terms at the time of checkups, we are saying, "Your body is special and it's your own. You don't need to allow anyone to invade it without a good reason."

I try to demonstrate this early in infancy. In my recent book *Touchpoints* I describe in detail how I approach a nine-month-old infant who is in the midst of stranger awareness, guarding vigilantly against potential intrusion. I examine a child this age in a parent's lap and the few extra minutes that I spend are an investment for the future. At a year, I start with a doll, then the parent, before placing the stethoscope on a child's chest, or the otoscope in an ear.

The child sees me demonstrate each of the procedures that are a part of the checkup. The visit becomes a learning experience. Children can experience each step via the doll, the parent, and can then finally allow me to examine them. This pays off later. I remember one two-and-a-half-year-old who came to my office for an earache. He sat compliantly in his father's lap, turning his head one way then the other for my otoscope. He opened his mouth wide for my flashlight. When we'd finished this exam, I was about ready to give his father my diagnosis. To my surprise, he lifted his shirt as if to remind me to listen to his heart and lungs. Over the preceding two years, I had spent perhaps twenty extra minutes letting him see what we were about to do on each visit.

He had learned to trust and cooperate with me over this short time, and this was our reward.

How could I turn Max down? If my grandson and I could explain in simple terms each step in a pediatric visit, couldn't we offer Max and his peers a reason to cooperate with these visits? We would try to understand what it means to a child to be undressed, to be examined with instruments that look into you, as though to see the "badness" you are trying to hide. "Why do my parents want me to go in for checkups? What are they trying to find?" This reluctance to being exposed is universal. Together we've tried to explain the reasons in terms small children can understand.

Parents can do a great deal to prepare a child for a doctor's or hospital visit. Our research some years ago at Children's Hospital in Boston demonstrated that children whose parents prepared them before admission for major surgery recovered significantly better. If parents showed them the oxygen tent, the surgical gowns, talked with them about the invasive procedures they could anticipate, the children's chances for survival after cardiac surgery were significantly increased. Children prepared in this way would even cough on demand after surgery, even though it hurt, to clear their lungs. This made a difference in their recovery. We carried this research on to other planned surgical admissions. When parents prepared their children for the steps they'd go through, the chil-

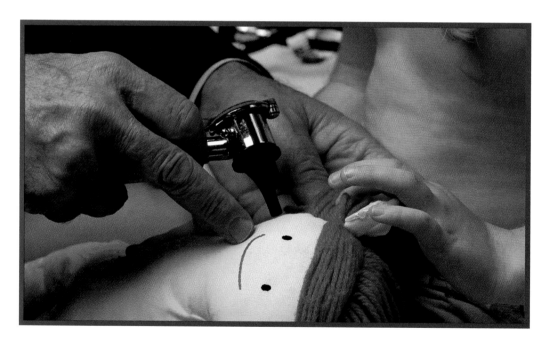

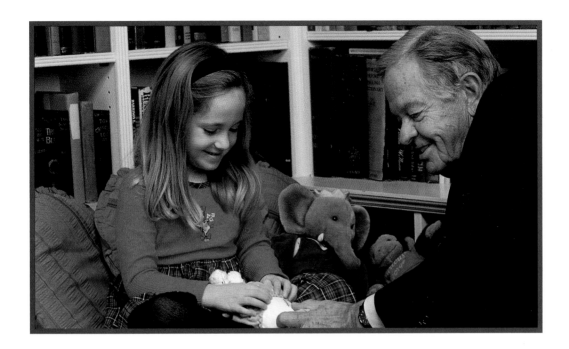

dren's cooperation in the hospital was significantly increased. Hospital stays were shortened. Recovery was more rapid. Their reactions at home were reduced—less bed-wetting, fewer fears at night, fewer school refusals. When parents share with a child such a potentially frightening experience as surgery, they are saying, "I'll be there with you, no matter what. You and I can face it together." This means to the child, "We can lick the pain and scary feelings that may come." The surgery becomes a shared learning experience.

Preparing a child for a regular checkup is just as important. "Tomorrow, we are going to see your doctor. Do you remember her (or him)? She certainly will remember you, for she keeps all those notes about you. She remembers your earache, and your wheezes last fall. Do you remember how she helped you get well? She remembers that you were afraid to go to first grade, but you did it! And look at you now. You're one of the best readers in the class. She'll be so proud. She remembers when you didn't know how to catch a ball, and now you're on the team. She knows all this because she's your doctor."

When a small child becomes frightened about coming to see me for a checkup, it's worth postponing the examination part. I ask his parents to bring him in several times before we actually examine him. The first time, I just say, "Hello. I want to be your doctor and your friend." The second time, I try to get him to get down off his mother's lap and to accept a small present for coming.

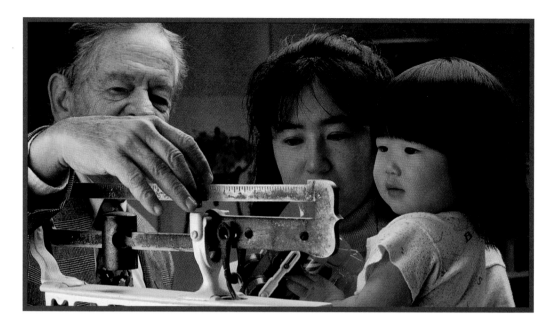

The third time I ask him to come around the corner of my desk for the present. On the fourth visit, I wear my stethoscope as I hand him the present in my office. Each time, I've let him know that I understand his fear, and that I want to be his doctor and his friend. By the next visit, he will be ready to be examined.

Talking about the visit gives a chance to ask questions. With this book, you can remind your child of the ingredients of the visit—the undressing, the stethoscope, the scales, and checking of all parts of the child's body. Remember that these steps are intrusive. Talking about them can detoxify them. You can share your own feelings. "I hate it when I get examined at my doctor's office, too. I'm always afraid he'll find something wrong with me. I forget that that's why I'm going to see him. If he finds anything, he and I can fix it together. After I've left his office, I feel so good. I hope you will, too."

When it's time to examine their bellies, I ask children to climb up on my examining table by themselves. Meanwhile, I can observe their muscles and their coordination. But also, they feel so proud to show me their ability. Then, when they lie down, they're not so worried. They are in control.

"Will I have to have a shot? I hate shots." (And children hate crying about them.) You can answer honestly, "I don't know in advance because I don't keep a record of them. But the doctor does. He knows when you need to have a booster shot so you won't get any of the diseases that could hurt you. If you do need one, I'll ask him to let me be there with you, to hold you and help you with it. You don't need to be brave. He knows how everyone hates shots. Go ahead and cry. He'll understand."

I ask parents to hold their small children when a shot is necessary. As soon as it's done, they are to dance around the room. It doesn't cut out the pain of the shot, but it does distract them from it. Still, the kids often look back at me as though they are saying, "You dirty guy! You hurt me!" Afterward, I like to give them a reward for being as brave as they've been. Some children bring in their toy doctor's kits to give me a shot while I'm preparing theirs. We both yell.

I've always given my own shots, for I feel that children should associate me with both the good and the bad. And maybe they'll see that even the shots are a way of protecting them from illnesses.

There are other ways to prepare a child that will make it easier for both the child and the doctor. What about ear exams? I find that I can't see eardrums unless the wax is out of the canal. Earwax piles up automatically in our ears. If you can put hydrogen peroxide in each ear at night for two or three days before you come in, it is likely to bubble the wax free, and the ear exam can be 100 percent more effective, and quicker.

What about the throat exam? The whole family can practice opening mouths wide. Then I won't need to use a tongue depressor. I can see the throat without one. If that doesn't work, you can hold the child in your lap with a full nelson, and I can get into her mouth and out in five seconds. She won't have time to mind it.

All these maneuvers ahead of time prepare children. They may not be eager to come in, but they'll be prepared. Some children get to feel right at home. I once made the mistake of leaving eight-year-old twins alone in my office briefly. When I returned, they were leaping from my examining table to my desk, yelling, "Batman!"

Please don't ever say to your children, "Don't cry," or "Don't be afraid." When you tell a child not to cry, you are opening the floodgates. And don't say, "You'll just love it," either. Of course she won't love it, but she'll master it. After it's over, she'll be proud. Let her know that you are, too.

The greatest compliment I have had came from a four-year-old waiting in my office. When I came out, she saw me and called, "Dr. B., I'm here! When is it my time?" Another time I was listening to two five-year-olds who were playing in my waiting room. They began to argue. "He's my doctor." "No, he's mine. He likes me!" Parents will understand what a triumph this is—for them, for the doctor, and above all, for the child.

My old patients now come in with their own children. Thirty years later, they remember the fish tank, the rock collection, the lollipop drawer. They feel a closeness with me that is unique. We respect each other. They know how proud I am of their successes, and of the responsibility for their own health that they have assumed. We became a team early, and they remember it. By starting with a simple explanation of a checkup visit, you as a parent can prepare your child to be ready for such a relationship. Perhaps this book will help. Above all, remember, it is your child's visit, your child's doctor.

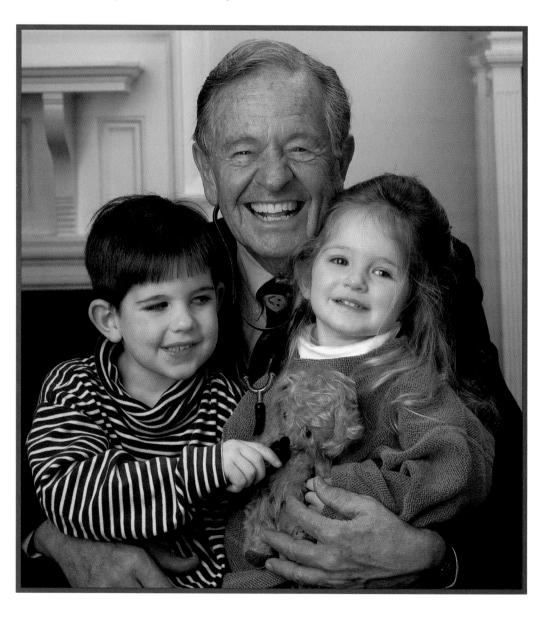

Sample Questions for Parents to Ask

The following questions are just examples of the kinds of concerns parents bring to their pediatricians or nurse practioners. Do not worry whether a question is awkward or inappropriate. No one knows your child better than you do. If something worries you about your child, the doctor should know. You might jot down your questions ahead of time so that you will remember them even if your child is wailing or climbing the walls.

How's he doing?
Is she gaining enough weight (or too much)? (Where is she on the growth chart?)
What should he be eating now? (He won't eat vegetables.)
Should she take vitamins?
How much sleep does he need?
Is there a way to avoid colds? Earaches?
When should I start potty training?
How should I treat small cuts?
What do I do if she won't take pills or other medicines?
What if he turns blue when he has a tantrum?
When should she start talking?
How do I know if he's hyperactive? (He's driving me crazy.)
How do I know if she's depressed? (She seems sad to me.)
How do I teach him responsibility? (I want him to do family chores.)
How can I teach her manners?
How can I stop him from biting his brother?
How can I help her make friends? (She is very shy.)
How can I motivate him? (His teacher says he is lazy.)
How involved should I be at her school to show that I care about her schoolwork?
How can I get him to do his homework without a fight every day?
How do I prepare her when I have to go off on a trip?
How do I prepare him for the death of a grandpa, cat, or schoolmate?
How do I keep her safe from possible sex abuse?
Should I worry about his nightmares?
How much TV should she watch?

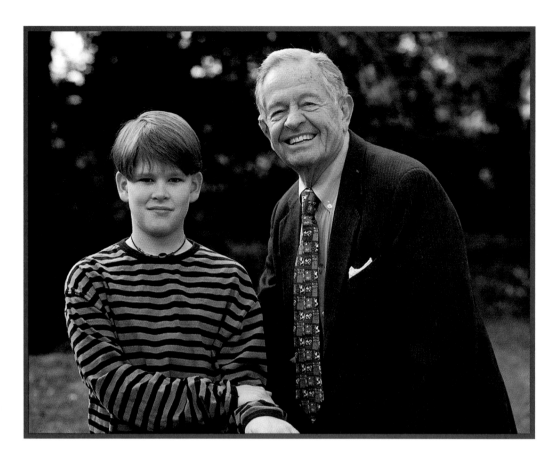

T. Berry Brazelton, M.D., Professor of Pediatrics Emeritus at Harvard Medical School, has cared for two generations of children in his Cambridge, Massachusetts, practice. While parents around the world have relied on his books, including *Infants and Mothers, To Listen to a Child,* and *Touchpoints, Going to the Doctor* is his first book for children, the audience dearest to his heart. Dr. Brazelton is the father of four children and the grandfather of four.

Alfred Womack, Dr. Brazelton's oldest grandchild, attends the Working Together Program at the Fitzgerald School in Cambridge. He enjoys drawing and illustrated this book when he was eight and nine years old. Now eleven, Alfred also likes swimming and being outdoors with his family on Cape Cod.

Sam Ogden—the father of Evan, two years old and one of the models in this book—is best known for portrait, magazine, and scientific photography. One of his recent projects was a marathon of photography for *24 Hours in Cyberspace.*